MANAGING PAIN IN SPORT

MANAGING PAIN IN SPORT

© P2P Publishing Ltd 2008

A CIP catalogue record for this book is available from the British Library.

Printed by: PLP Commercial Printers
Impressions House, 3-7 Mowlem Street, London E2 9HE

Published by P2P Publishing Ltd

Registered office: 33-41 Dallington, London, EC1V 0BB
Tel: 0845 450 6402
Registered number: 06014651

ISBN: 978-1-905096-34-3

Publisher Jonathan A. Pye
Editor Sam Bordiss
Designer The Flying Fish Studios Ltd
Illustration Viv Mullett

CONTENTS

Contributors

Louis Gifford is a Fellow of the Chartered Society of Physiotherapy and has been writing and lecturing on pain for over 18 years. As well as working in his own private practice in Cornwall he lectures extensively in the UK, Europe and worldwide and currently edits the Physiotherapy Pain Association's book series entitled *Topical Issues in Pain*.

Andrew Hamilton BSc, MRSC, trained as a chemist and is consultant to the fitness industry and an experienced science writer. He's now editor of *Peak Performance*.

Australian-born **Matt Lancaster** relocated to the United Kingdom in 2000 and is currently employed by the English Institute of Sport as lead physiotherapist for the London region.

Stephen Robson has worked in his own private practice and sports injury clinic in Northumberland for ten years. He writes and lectures on pain and has been a physiotherapist to the British Olympic squad and Royal Yachting Association for seven years.

From the editor

No pain, no gain… Pain is temporary, winning is forever… everyone has heard a pain euphemism while participating in sport. It's part and parcel of the fun. Except in the most part, pain is not that much fun. It means you've damaged a part of your all-important body, it means you can't compete to your best, and worst of all it hurts!

Having played rugby as my primary sport for ten years or so, and being a competitive alpha male with a tendency to go gung-ho, I have experienced more than my fair share of pain. Unfortunately reading through these articles has made the pain even worse, simply because I've realised I could have saved myself a lot of anguish throughout my playing days!

The opening chapter is styled as a Q&A, with painful questions relieved by comprehensive answers. The second and third chapters are linked, the first part explaining a revolutionary approach to chronic injury focusing on the management of pain. The second part contains two case studies, a young rugby player and an older golfer, implementing the theories of the first part. Finally the fourth chapter investigates the dangers of non-steroidal anti-inflammatory drugs, or painkillers.

If ever there was a report to help people, it's this one!

Sam Bordiss
Editor

PAIN

Q and A: Pain and gain – how athletes can manage and overcome pain?

'Pain is inevitable, but suffering is optional.' So goes a well-known but anonymous quote. For many athletes, pain is a normal everyday experience and success is often achieved in spite of pain. But what's the best strategy for coping with and overcoming pain and how can athletes distinguish between benign and potentially damaging pain?

How do some people shrug off a painful injury?

Remember that following an acute injury, such as an ankle sprain, pain receptors are first stimulated by the mechanical stress and strain placed upon the tissue. 'Inflammatory soup' soon floods the tissue leading to peripheral sensitisation. Several hours later, similar chemicals will also lead to spinal modulation[1]. Pain and sensitivity to movement and pressure increase over a period of a few hours; the time between the transition from the original mechanical pain (which may pass) to the maximum sensitised state may provide athletes with a 'window of opportunity' to shrug off their pain and continue competing.

However, this mechanism is probably only the tip of the iceberg. When you are totally focused on your opponent, or consumed by the contest, supraspinal and spinal modulation may act to inhibit the transmission or limit the awareness of the pain signal[1]. We've all heard stories of sportsmen and women who have continued despite an injury which (theoretically) should have caused them to stop: a boxer with a broken hand, rugby players with torn ligaments, a long jumper with a strained hamstring *etc*. In the cut and thrust of competition, the pain system can 'shut the gate', and athletes are able to continue in spite of injured tissue[2]. However, once your attention is drawn back to the acute pain (particularly following competition), awareness of the pain becomes strong again, especially if this also coincides with an increase in peripheral and spinal modulation.

So, should you ignore pain and try to shrug off an injury? Acute sensitisation is a normal, helpful process to encourage you to stop using the injured tissue and avoid further damage[3]. It might be helpful to ask yourself the three questions in the box below.

There are a few other questions, which are perhaps even more important. We'll get to these later. But remember, acute pain usually occurs for a good reason. It makes sense to seek professional advice as soon as you can. Sometimes people can overcome acute pain and continue to compete, but that doesn't necessarily make it a wise decision!

The three Cs

- Can you cope with the pain?
- Are you able to contribute a meaningful performance?
- What are the consequences of continuing?

How can two athletes with the same injury experience different pain?

Studies have confirmed that people respond differently to similar levels of painful stimulation[2]. Differences exist not just in our individual sensitivity to a painful stimulus, but also in our perception of pain and how we display it. Pain is individual, even when the stimulus is not, but while we cannot know exactly what someone else is experiencing, our brains undergo quite similar activity when confronted with someone else's pain[4]. This is the basis for empathy and acknowledging someone's pain is normal and important.

Our individual sensitivity to pain is in part explained by our genetic makeup[5-7], while studies involving twins have shown that learned behaviours are also important[8]. Again, the division of pain into real and mental is unhelpful and the variation in pain between two athletes with the same injury lies at all levels of the pain system. Even for the same athlete, pain sensitivity varies under different circumstances, and perhaps not surprisingly, can become significantly less during competition[9].

It's also worth noting that different groups in society may have significantly different pain responses, and this applies within sport. A study performed 40 years ago demonstrated that contact sport athletes could tolerate experimental acute pain for longer than non-contact athletes, while both groups could tolerate more acute pain than non-athletes[9].

Pain sensitivity may also be different in different people at different times; the way athletes display that they are in pain can vary, both between individuals and also between groups of athletes from different sports. It might be an extreme example, but imagine a footballer who could potentially be rewarded with a penalty responding to the pain from a kick in the shin. Now, assuming the tissue damage is equivalent, think about the same incident involving a Thai kick boxer who is in the middle of a title fight. Get the idea?!

Why do some pains seem to last forever?

During ongoing or chronic pain, adaptive changes at all levels of the pain system often outlast their usefulness in helping us protect injured tissues. Movements and pressures that would otherwise be normal continue to cause pain long after the risk of further injury has passed and often even once the tissue has essentially healed.

Examining possible tissue damage remains important when considering ongoing or recurrent pains, but a broader approach is required to address an athlete's fear and anxiety about their ongoing pain and help them return to their sport. Focusing too much attention on pain can actually increase pain[2]. It is probably more helpful to concentrate on working hard to

The dos and don'ts of pain and performance

As explained above, everyone responds differently to pain stimuli, responses that may vary according to social and emotional environments and even expectation. However, here are a few tips that all athletes and coaches should bear in mind:

DO

- **Acknowledge pain** – Pain is pain. It is not 'physical or mental'. Coaches and other team members should understand that showing empathy is normal and helpful;
- **Seek professional advice** – Consult a sports doctor or physiotherapist for any acute, ongoing or recurrent pain;
- **Recover and rehabilitate** – Focus on allowing the tissue time to heal and work to become strong and fit again.

DON'T

- **Be too concerned** – Too much focus and attention on pain is counterproductive to sporting performance;
- **Fear pain** – Hearsay stories of similar pains ending careers are unhelpful. Pain is a normal part of sport; don't let it become a catastrophe;
- **Punish or reward** – Being angry at or ignoring athletes is as unhelpful as being over attentive. Remain positive, interested and constructive.

strengthen the tissues at a sensible rate, regain normal fitness and aim to return to training.

Providing an appropriate environment for people to overcome ongoing pain is important and not always easy in sport. Coaches or team-mates who are angry at or ignore athletes with ongoing pain may contribute further to those athletes avoiding the very things that will help them return to full activity (such as a rehabilitation programme), and generate further anxiety that doesn't help either[10]. Getting this balance right and remaining positive is therefore important. People who develop an exaggerated, negative mindset towards their ongoing pain have been shown to experience both increased pain and emotional distress[11]. Pain is a normal part of sport but the right mental approach can prevent it from becoming a catastrophe.

Does this mean it is OK to ignore ongoing pain? Well, it's not quite that simple. Once again consider the three Cs. Any pain that has been present for more than a week or so, or keeps returning periodically is worth getting checked out by a professional who can not only assess for tissue damage but can also understand your pain and hopefully point you in the right direction before the maladaptive changes to your nervous system become entrenched.

Why are some people able to compete, seemingly regardless of pain, while others struggle to overcome even a minor niggle?

Although pain (especially acute pain) is related to tissue damage, this damage alone is not sufficient to explain pain fully. Pain is not just a sensation but results from the interaction between sensory inputs and brain processes, such as emotion and conscious thought. And pain is individual, not just to you as an athlete, but also to the time, circumstance and environment you find yourself in. Within the mechanics of the pain system, individual variation and modulation occur subconsciously, which helps to answer this question.

To ultimately address the relationship between pain and sport however, it is necessary to consider one further aspect of pain: your own 'personal values'. We've already considered the three Cs as a guide to considering how to act in the presence of pain; however, as anyone involved with sport knows, making decisions about athletes in pain is often a judgement call. The three C questions only have meaning if we add a further, more personal line of questioning:

- Am I prepared to cope?
- How important is contributing a worthwhile performance to me?
- Am I prepared to suffer the consequences?

Having a pain killing injection two days before an Olympic final, regardless of the risks, would seem quite a reasonable thing to do for most elite athletes if it was the only way they were able to compete. Under similar circumstances, few casual joggers would agree to the same injection just days before a fun run. Entering a boxing ring, running 100 miles a week or crashing into a rugby scrum is not for everyone. Some people can continually and repeatedly overcome pain for the sake of their sport because they are prepared to. Sometimes they are rewarded with success, and sometimes, despite their desire to cope and contribute, their body succumbs to the consequences. Winners and heroes overcome pain sometimes. Losers often try and fail. Perhaps the most successful sports people are those who best understand the relationship between pain and performance: they are prepared to overcome pain, but make wise, informed decisions about when it is worthwhile trying to do so.

Matt Lancaster

References

1. *Brain 2003; 126:1079-1091*

2. *Trends in Pharmacological Sciences 2005; 26(3):125-130*

3. *Topical Issues in Pain 1 (CNS Press) 1998; 45-57*

4. *Pain 2006; 125:5-9*

5. *Human Molecular Genetics 2005; 14(1):135-143*

6. *Proc Natl Acad Sci 1999; 96:7744-7751*

7. *Pain Practice 2005; 5(4):341-348*

8. *Arthritis & Rheumatism 2004; 51(2):160-167*

9. *Sport Jrnl 2003; 6(2)*

10. *Pain 2005; 113:155-159*

11. *Clinical Jrnl Pain 2001; 17:52-64*

PART ONE -
A revolutionary approach
to chronic injury

*Injury and pain are a competitive athlete's worst nightmare,
scuppering even the best-laid training plans. And when injuries
become chronic, they can destroy confidence and even end athletic
careers. But a revolution is taking place in our understanding of
pain, which has profound implications for the treatment and
rehabilitation of many chronic injuries. As explained in the first of
this two-part series, it's time to throw away many of our existing
preconceptions about pain and injury*

The trouble with pain is that it is normal to hurt. In fact to be
more specific, pain is an evolutionary masterpiece that protects
us from injury by alerting us to actual or perceived threat or
damage to our tissues. However, until recently all of the various
orthodox and alternative branches of medicine have understood
very little about pain and consequently how to treat it *(see 'The
history of pain', overleaf)*.

We now know that pain is a multi-dimensional amalgamation
and integration of biological, psychological and sociological
factors. In the same way that differences in our individual
biology, psychology and social circumstances make us
individual and who we are as people, these factors also
influence our experience of pain. To understand why this is so,
we first need to understand some basic facts about pain

Surprising facts about pain
Pain involves complex neural circuits *(see diagram, page 19)*
from the tissues of the body into the central nervous

system/brain and back out again. Therefore, all pain involves the brain. Pain influences the brain, the brain influences the mind (a convenient collective term for those states of brain activity involving awareness), and the mind and brain combine to produce a response. Hence how an individual interprets and reacts to pain has a very powerful influence over the pain and its outcome.

Sensory information is processed and interpreted by your central nervous system. This requires highly complex brain functions involving scrutiny of past experiences, knowledge,

The history of pain

The last ten years have seen more progress in our understanding of pain than the entire preceding history of medicine. This explosion of 'pain knowledge' has been, in medical terms, equivalent to discovering that the world is round and not flat.

Before this recent period of 'pain discovery', treatment for painful conditions was largely based on tradition, faith and guesswork. A vast array of orthodox and alternative pain treatments became available throughout this period and many continue to be used today. Medical doctors, physiotherapists, osteopaths and chiropractors right through to crystal therapists have all presented their theories and philosophies regarding their particular approach to treating pain.

Because these professions emerged before the current scientific evidence was available, and at a time when there was little if any evidence on which to base treatment approaches, the result was the development of therapeutic approaches based on theories and philosophies rather than reliable scientific evidence. On reflection it is probably unsurprising to learn that throughout this time the success of treatments for painful conditions has in scientific terms been modest to disastrous.

Until recently many of the theories behind pain treatments were based around the work of a 17th century French philosopher named René Descartes. Descartes believed that the mind and body operated separately and as such, pain signals followed a single pathway straight from the damaged body part to be registered consciously in the brain.

It has taken almost four centuries for medical science to establish enough evidence to know that Descartes was wrong. We now know that the brain is wholly involved in the processing of pain and is actually the major control centre when it comes to pain. Finding this out has been hugely important in our current understanding of pain and how to treat it.

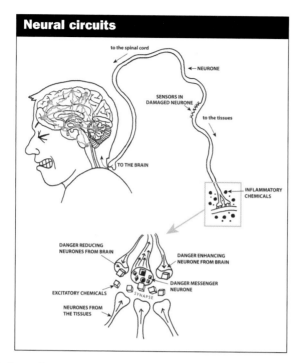

Neural circuits

beliefs, culture, past successful behaviours and successful behaviours observed in others[1].

So for example, take exactly the same type of injury occurring at the Achilles tendon of an office worker and a professional footballer. The office worker may interpret this injury as nothing more than an irritating discomfort; however, in a footballer this same injury may be interpreted as a threat to their fitness, career and livelihood and thus 'negative reaction' or appraisal can lead to more pain and even a slowing of recovery rate.

Pain is not an isolated reaction in the tissues that are injured or that hurt – *ie* you can't feel anything without a brain (no brain – no pain!). There is also a psychological reaction in everyone who feels pain and this drives subsequent behaviour, affecting outcomes. For example, a runner who experiences pain in the back of their leg while running may respond to this pain in the following way:

• 'I've never had pain like this before' (past experience);

- 'Sciatica causes pain down the back of the leg but so does a hamstring strain' (knowledge);
- 'I've heard that you can't really get rid of sciatica' (beliefs);
- 'I won't say anything to my training partner – I'll keep a stiff upper lip and just keep running' (culture);
- 'Maybe I should see my doctor, those pills he gave me for my calf pain last year really helped' (past successful behaviours);
- 'My brother went to see that physiotherapist in town and he sorted his hamstring strain out' (past successful behaviours observed in others).

The outcome in this example is that the runner makes an appointment to see the physiotherapist – *ie* a behaviour driven by the psychological reaction to the leg pain.

More suprising facts

Pain is very commonly not a reliable witness to the extent of injury or tissue damaged. For example, sciatica (a condition that may disable an athlete) can lead to huge amounts of pain experienced from a tiny area of tissue injury. At the opposite extreme, spinal disc bulges/herniations are known to occur and exist without causing any pain whatsoever[2,3].

In fact, most if not all of us have experienced examples of tissue damage occurring without pain. For example, have you ever wondered how you could have failed to feel pain from that bruise or cut you didn't even notice was there until you discovered it while showering?

Bruises and cuts are obvious signs of tissue damage yet often do not produce pain at the time of injury. In these circumstances the central nervous system has received the tissue injury signals from the cut or bruise, scrutinised them and decided that the area will recover without necessitating any changes to your behaviour. Therefore no pain is required to make you rest, limp *etc* (*ie* behave differently) to help allow the tissue to heal.

Contrary to popular belief, most injuries affect multiple structures, eg back strains. The idea of a single tissue culprit being the source of pain may be untenable[2].

Injury and disease processes obviously change the state of tissues. However, if pain is a feature of these processes, it usually starts as a result of mechanical and chemical influences in the tissues activating nociceptors (nociceptors are nerve fibres normally dedicated to sensing intense or threatening stimuli). For example, an acutely twisted ankle or calf tear results in mechanically derived damage to the tissues involved, followed by inflammation and the subsequent chemical irritation of local nociceptors.

Stopping the activity of the nociceptors that serve the area of tissue damage at a time near the onset of pain, using agents such as local anaesthetic, will completely obliterate the pain (it stops the dominoes toppling – see below). Stopping or curtailing inflammation may dull nociceptive activity enough to take out a proportion of the pain too. This is how non-steroidal anti-inflammatory drugs such as ibuprofen work.

Injury or irritation of peripheral nerves and nerve roots (the bulbous part of the peripheral nerve just outside of the spinal cord) can also be a starting point for pain, eg acute sciatica. One commonly recognised initial cause of sciatica is that of spinal discs herniating/bulging out onto the sciatic nerve. However, surgically removing or altering the offending disc will often fail to stop an irritated nerve from causing pain, even though the disc may have initiated the process[2,4].

Domino effect

The neurophysiological reasons for this are extensive and beyond the scope of this article. However, you can think of the ongoing process of pain as akin to a 'domino effect'. Imagine a line of dominoes, where the first domino in line represents tissue injury (disc, nerve, ligament, muscle *etc*), the second represents the nociceptor and further dominoes represent all of the subsequent nerve connections right up into the brain.

If the first domino is toppled (signifying tissue injury), this causes each domino in turn to topple all of the way down the line, just like a sequence of nerve signals from the tissue going up to the brain.

Hopefully, you can also see from this representation that, just like pain, even if you stand the first domino back up again (the equivalent of surgically removing or treating the offending tissue) this would not stop or reverse the rest of the dominoes toppling, and therefore the signal can still continue onwards to register as pain in the brain.

These signals can continue to reverberate within the central nervous system long after tissues have healed. This is part of the reason why many people, including athletes, still continue to experience pain even after they have undergone surgery to remove injured tissues like discs or cartilage, or after they have received treatments to help injured tissues to heal.

We now understand that most persistent, ongoing pain associated with an injury is driven and maintained by mechanisms and changes that occur within the 'circuitry' of the central nervous system as a result of injury and that this is often not a sign of any active ongoing tissue injury. In simple terms, it's quite possible to have ongoing pain without any actual tissue damage and therefore 'hurt does not always mean harm' in the same way that 'harm does not always mean hurt'.

This helps to explain why the treatment of chronic pain resulting from injury is so frequently unsuccessful; the original injury may already have healed and it's the circuitry of the central nervous system that really needs attention.

Maladaptive and chronic pain

All this means there's good news for many athletes with chronic injuries; firstly, hurt does not necessarily equate to harm' and secondly, there is such a thing as maladaptive (biologically unhelpful) pain. You can think of maladaptive pain in terms of 'active aberrant pain circuitry' that remains switched on in the central nervous system long after tissues have healed.

Unlike 'new' acute pain, ongoing maladaptive pain does not help recovery because it doesn't produce behavioural changes that allow healing. This is because the tissues involved have already healed to their maximal potential long ago and therefore the remaining pain is 'useless'.

When pain is not benign

Although most chronic pain is benign, we must always be aware that a very small but significant percentage of people with pain do have serious underlying disease or pathology causing it. For example, although it's extremely rare, chronic pain could be an indication of tumour, infection or fracture. Screening for serious disorders is a highly skilled part of the examination process, and a detailed history, physical examination (and sometimes a referral to other medical experts) are essential to rule out more sinister causes of pain.

It is therefore imperative when seeking help for painful conditions that whoever you are consulting is properly medically qualified and trained to do this and your physiotherapist should be state-registered as a minimum. Physiotherapists who are members of the Physiotherapy Pain Association (PPA) have a specific interest in treating pain, and have often done additional post-graduate training in this area. More information is available at www.pponline.co.uk.

Hence the problems with therapy approaches that over-focus on finding a specific source of pain – fine for fixing a car but far too simple for fixing complex human pain states. For example, focusing on joints by manipulating or mobilising them, or on muscles by strengthening or stabilising them loses sight of the bigger picture. The source of much of the long-lasting pain associated with chronic injury is likely to be in the central nervous system – not in the tissues.

The tissues that hurt may only play a small part in the pain, if any. This makes continued therapeutic focus on those tissues that hurt, at best, only moderately effective and possibly ineffective or detrimental.

Implications of maladaptive pain

The new understanding of pain, particularly chronic maladaptive pain, is revealing major shortcomings in conventional treatment therapies (where a specific tissue is treated). For example, as time passes, the original cause of the pain may become irrelevant. Thus, while a spinal disc injury may precipitate a back pain or sciatica, as time passes its state may be far less relevant to the pain.

It's also incorrect to reason that if a therapy targeted at a particular structure is successful in alleviating the pain, then that structure has to be responsible for the pain. For example, if a therapist mobilises the joints of a patient's neck and the patient's elbow pain improves, the traditional reasoning assumes the neck joints as a likely or potential source of the pain because this is the level where the nerves to the elbow emerge from the spine. However, pressure on the foot (reflexology for example) or ear lobe (some forms of acupuncture) could have achieved the same thing, and sometimes does if the therapy can be set up to be acceptable in the eyes of the patient.

In the same way, surgical removal of spinal disc material with a subsequent alleviation of pain does not necessarily mean that the disc material was the source of the pain. There are many examples in medical literature where surgeons have performed exploratory surgery alone on the low backs of patients who, following their surgery, have reported relief of their back pain and sciatica. In plain English, anaesthetise a patient, cut them open, dig around a bit, have a good look, find nothing of interest, sew them back up again – and about 40% will be completely relieved of their symptoms[5].

Effective pain treatment

We also know that if pain changes quickly with treatment, the most responsible explanation for the mechanism of the effect is that it is down to changes in the processing of information in the central nervous system. However, treatments for pain are likely to be much more effective in both the short and long term if they are based on the biological and psychosocial factors that science has identified as being integral to everyone's experience of pain. Remarkably, it seems that pain can often be treated from anywhere in the body – any of a number of techniques that successfully interact biologically or psychologically with a patient can be effective in modulating pain.

In the second of this two-part series, we illustrate how this radical 'biopsychosocial' approach to pain can be applied in practice to treat chronic injuries in athletes. Two case studies are presented, involving successful treatment of chronic neck and arm pain in an elite golfer, and hamstring pain in an elite rugby player. There'll also be information on how to spot the tell-tale signs of neurologically produced pain, and how to distinguish it from acute pain associated with actual tissue damage. Finally we'll discuss how this new, evidence-based approach is forcing us to re-evaluate some of the current treatment approaches to chronic neck, shoulder and back pain, such as core stability training, and why some of these current approaches may even be counterproductive in the longer term.

Stephen Robson and Louis Gifford

References

1. Gifford L, Topical Issues In Pain, NOI Press, Falmouth, 45-56, 1998

2. Gifford L, In Touch, 97: 3-9, 2001

3. Robson S, PPA News, 16: 12-17, Dec 2003

4. Robson S, Topical Issues In Pain, 5th edn. CNS Press, Falmouth (in press), 2005

5. Gifford L, Topical Issues In Pain 4, CNS Press, Falmouth, 19-75, 2002

PART TWO:
The biopsychosocial method of chronic injury rehabilitation

In the previous chapter we discussed the current scientific evidence surrounding pain and how pain can become persistent and maladaptive despite prior healing of the tissue injuries that initially cause the pain. This second part explains exactly how the 'biopsychosocial' approach can be used to rehabilitate chronic injuries

The conventional approach to treating pain and injury will almost certainly include a biomedical assessment, *ie* an assessment of the state of the tissues that may be involved with each person's pain. This is the part of clinical examination that most people are familiar with, involving physical testing of things like joint movements, muscle power, reflexes *etc*. Good biomedical assessment tries to determine the following:

- Is there any evidence that might indicate serious injury or disease?;
- Is the problem a 'common syndrome' with a well-defined natural history? For example, frozen shoulder is a common syndrome that can be predicted in terms of its longevity and prognosis;
- Is the nervous system competent? This requires skilled and appropriate neurological testing;
- Are the tissues that hurt or that may be responsible for the pain strong enough to be progressively loaded?;
- What pain mechanisms are operating and are they adaptive/helpful or maladaptive/unhelpful? *(see box, overleaf).*

What kind of pain have I got?

Knowing whether the pain associated with an injury is adaptive (helpful) or maladaptive (unhelpful) is critical to determining how to progress and rehabilitate that injury. Although a proper diagnosis requires a skilled and qualified physiotherapist, there are some useful pointers:

Adaptive pain

- Produces behaviours that promote recovery and healing. A sprained calf muscle is usually very sore to walk on the next morning because the pain is demanding that you look after the muscle while the first (inflammatory) stages of the repair process get underway;
- After a day or two the initial pain of movement subsides as you move the tissues more and more, indicating that the healing tissue likes some movement;
- Move too much and the tissue gets sore again and demands more rest;
- Rest too long and the discomfort can also get you to move once more – ie adaptive pain makes you stop a bit, and go a bit – just what healing requires.

NB. If tissues have a history of injury, or are arthritic, some adaptive pain may have to be accepted. However, these tissues can still be rehabilitated to become very strong and capable of high performance given appropriate functional graded exercises and adequate warm-ups on the day.

Maladaptive pain

- Often out of all proportion to the actual tissue damage done (eg the nerve pain described in Sam's case – see case history on page 10);
- Pain persists long after the initial injury, even though the healing phase has been completed;
- Pain is the problem rather than the actual tissues that contain the pain, which may be just weak, deconditioned or contain modest scar tissue, none of which make pain inevitable;
- May often require a carefully graded, acceptable and activity-relevant approach to strengthen the tissues and fully rehabilitate the athlete.

The biopsychosocial approach differs, however, in that it also focuses on psychological and social factors *(see box, page 31)*, which have been shown to be vital considerations in predicting the outcome from a musculoskeletal pain problem – even stronger predictors of outcome than any individual biomedical measures.

For example, an athlete with a significant disc protrusion causing back pain and sciatica will not necessarily have a poor outcome, but if he or she believes that any activity that provokes the slightest discomfort should be avoided and as a result rests completely, the likelihood is that it will be harder to return to sport and normal activities than had the athlete confronted their problem and tried to keep going. In short, the outcome for any sportsman or woman suffering from pain and injury is hugely determined by how they interpret and react to the situation they are in.

Clinicians also have a huge impact on how well patients cope and how they recover, most especially early on. For example, advice and therapy that creates fear of movement, or fear of biomechanical or structural weakness, or that focuses too much on pain at the expense of function, has enormous negative connotations. However, an approach that appropriately reassures the patient with evidence-based education, advice and functional rehabilitation can progressively restore their confidence, assist recovery and get them back to normal activity[1].

Biopsychosocial approach in action – case studies
The two case histories that follow are not meant to be prescriptive for the pain problems both of these athletes were facing. Instead they give some practical examples and ideas that can be helpful in the treatment and management of pain.

Johnny – an 18-year-old county and national rugby player
Johnny's problem started when he was 16 years old and playing rugby; during a sprint down the wing he felt a sharp pain in the back of his left thigh that immediately brought him to a halt. He was unable to continue playing and rested for a number of weeks with what he described as a 'torn hamstring'.

He gradually made a successful return to rugby but then experienced a further four recurrences of this pain. He had grown more and more concerned that his injury didn't seem to be progressing – in fact, if anything it was getting worse and he was able to do less and less rugby training as time went on. He had made big efforts to maintain his cardiovascular fitness by cycling and swimming regularly and was continuing to do his strength training in the gym, but avoided hamstring exercises because they hurt.

Initially, I spent considerable time talking to him and using the A, B, C, D, E, F & W approach *(see box, right)*, I discovered that he believed his hamstring was seriously damaged and that his pain was from further harm being caused to the hamstring every time he tried to use it. As a result he avoided any activity that caused the slightest reproduction of his pain. He also believed that he had poor 'core stability' and major 'muscle imbalance' around his low back, pelvis and lower limbs.

His behaviour had fluctuated between long periods of rugby training inactivity to a 'boom or bust' approach when he had moved straight from a period of relative inactivity and attempted to return to full training all at once. It emerged that his belief regarding his poor core stability and muscle imbalance was the result of a 'diagnosis' given to him by a physiotherapist looking after one of the squads he belonged to.

After two years of this problem he had lost the enjoyment he used to have for rugby and was worried about his future in the sport – so anxious he would constantly mentally check himself to see whether he could feel any pain at his hamstring. Although his mother and father were concerned about him, they had begun to show frustration at his poor recovery from this problem, and one of his coaches was convinced he was 'exaggerating the seriousness of his injuries'.

A biomedical examination revealed:
- He had exceptionally good muscle tone throughout his body and there was no obvious leg length inequality or asymmetry;
- Movements at his low back and hips were full and painless and neurological tests performed throughout both lower limbs were normal;
- Muscle length tests at both lower limbs did not reveal any shortening of the involved structures and indicated that his hamstring length and flexibility was excellent;
- Resisted manual muscle tests applied to the left hamstring indicated normal power but did reproduce his pain;

Psychosocial assessment

A psychosocial assessment is often logically carried out using the headings A, B, C, D, E, F and W[2]:
- **Attitudes and beliefs about pain.**
- **Behaviours;** how people respond to pain, what they avoid or have difficulty with and how they react and report their situation.
- **Compensation issues;** compensation, disputes, financial hassles and legal wrangles following injuries often create a lot of stress for people and certainly do not help.
- **Diagnosis and treatment issues;** what health professionals say to patients. For example, complicated medical language and diagnoses, conflicting diagnoses, explanations that create notions of physical weakness or long-term incapacity (you have the spine of a 70 year old), dramatic and unscientific explanations of injuries and pathology and 'salesmanlike' approaches to therapy that can falsely raise expectations of a 'quick and easy' cure.
- **Emotions;** chronic pain and injury can lead to increasing levels of distress, altered routines and habits, reduced social interaction and even clinical depression. Athletes experiencing pain should be involved in taking control and responsibility for their pain, which is often the start of improved fitness, self-esteem and the confidence to move forward.
- **Family;** family and friends can have a big impact on how individuals react towards their pain, sometimes reinforcing a 'be careful don't move' style of coping while at the same time taking away responsibilities and making the athlete feel hopeless and useless.
- **Work;** being engaged in both the physical and mental tasks of work are essential components for recovery. If you reduce or stop physical activity and work, you'll have nothing better to do than sit around and think about your pain all day every day. It is a sobering statistic that 90% of people who are 'off work' for six months or longer never return to full-time employment[3].

- Palpation at the midpoint of the hamstring evoked tenderness and further functional tests also reproduced his pain during running, jumping and hopping activities.

These findings did not indicate the possible presence of serious disease or injury, and we therefore proceeded to agree on a plan of management to address his problem. During our discussion I made efforts to point out all that was positive with his examination as well as those things that could be worked on to assist his recovery.

I also explained that his pain had become maladaptive and that it stemmed from a multi-dimensional biopsychosocial problem, which although involving powerful brain processing, was not 'psychosomatic' as had been suggested to him. I further pointed out that treatments that focus too much on single tissues or one part of the body system, for example the muscle system in the core stability approach, have yet to produce any compelling results in the clinical research trials that have been carried out[4,5].

Therapy problems

Although the concept of maladaptive pain is gradually gaining wider acceptance in physiotherapy, it is still a poorly understood concept, particularly in the field of sports therapy, where the focus tends to remain on some sort of tissue abnormality, muscle imbalance, joint tightness, trigger point or disordered movement pattern – to name a few. While these approaches may be helpful in some cases, they certainly are not if the end result is an over-focus on pain or on some unproven 'weakness' somewhere. Increased attention and anxiety about a structure or about a pain only serves to increase awareness and hence leads to increased pain.

In Johnny's case, not only was there no evidence that his core stability was poor, focusing on this perceived muscle imbalance only served to constantly direct his attention to the pain he was experiencing, increasing anxiety and therefore compounding the problem. Moreover, by constantly thinking about contracting his tranversus abdominis to try to combat this perceived instability, he was actually learning new and unnatural patterns of movement associated with the pain – exactly the opposite of what is required for 'thoughtless fearless movement'[6].

We also looked at how we could approach his rehabilitation avoiding the 'inactivity' or 'boom or bust' cycle by using an approach known as graded exposure. This involves gradually exposing patients to the very movements that are actively feared or avoided. Graded exposure requires that patients want to overcome their fear, understand that exercise will help the problem not hinder, and are willing to put in the effort and time.

The initial aim is to make each exercise simple, easy and achievable so that it doesn't produce pain (which can be demotivating) and the patient feels confident they can manage it. We initially identified a number of component movements (*ie* that are relevant to the feared and avoided movements/ activities) that could be improved in terms of their endurance, strength and quality. Easily achievable baselines were set as were the goal amounts for each exercise and Johnny worked through these diligently.

The specificity of his programme was constantly adjusted to achieve greater ranges of movement, increased and alternating speed of movements and improved muscle strength and endurance *(see box below for an example of this approach)*. The ultimate goal at all times was to restore 'thoughtless, fearless movement'. Normal movement does not have any fear, apprehension or thoughts associated with it, and restoring this state through graded exposure and careful exercise pacing often results in the ultimate success with rehabilitation. In Johnny's case, he made a sustained return to first class rugby three months later.

An example of graded exposure

Johnny had difficulty bending his right knee and moving his hip backwards against resistance without pain. We tried a number of different positions in which to perform these movements and found that standing was the one he liked best. His range of movement was full but there was some discomfort at the end of the movement when he actively bent his knee. We reduced the range of movement and looked at the middle part of his range and found this to be pain free and easy to perform.

We then added some resistance by attaching a light resistance latex exercise band around his lower leg above the ankle and he then attempted a number of repetitions that he felt would be easy and achievable. We reduced this number slightly and this was set as his baseline.

Having decided on a goal number of repetitions and sets, he worked through these at his own pace, gradually increasing to his goal amount. We then established new baselines and goals incorporating more resistance and increased range and speed of movement.

His exercises were then integrated and progressed into more functional activities such as running, bounding and hopping drills, where the focus was to develop his ability to alternate the speed and direction of movement so that his rehabilitation reflected the components of his sport. Later on in his rehabilitation we liaised directly with his coaches to carry these principles right through to his return to competitive rugby. The aim throughout was to help him to restore a state of 'thoughtless fearless movement'[6].

Sam – a 42-year-old elite golfer

Sam began experiencing right-sided neck, shoulder and arm pain, which had become much more severe and was now accompanied by occasional episodes of pins and needles over the arm. He was also aware that his right arm was getting weaker and his shoulder movement seemed to be getting progressively more restricted, which was now interfering with his golf swing.

The same assessment approach was used as previously described for Johnny. Psychosocial information gathered included a belief that his pain was harmful. He also has a close friend who was a former European golf tour professional and whose career was blighted and prematurely ended by 'a similar injury'.

Sam had largely avoided playing golf and had rarely practised over the previous three months. His GP had diagnosed a 'trapped nerve' after referring him for an MRI scan, which showed a disc prolapse affecting one of the nerves on the right side of his neck. His GP subsequently organised a referral to a neurosurgeon and told him that he would probably need an operation. Emotionally, Sam was very anxious about this diagnosis and the idea of surgery on his neck, as well as by his inability to play golf or to play freely with his children. He had continued going to work but was struggling with some jobs that involved lifting, reaching and stretching.

A biomedical examination revealed:

- He preferred to sit or stand with his head and neck flexed forwards (this position reduced his pain);
- His neck movements were painfully limited and increased his neck, shoulder and arm pain when he extended his head backwards or towards his right side;
- Neurological tests revealed that the nerves in the region were sensitive to being compressed and elongated;
- He also had weakness at the muscles of the right arm that are supplied by these same nerves. Functionally, he could not place his right arm behind his back or take it into the top of the back swing position of his golf swing.

I took time to explain my provisional diagnosis of pain coming from a peripheral nerve. Although this condition is often referred to as a 'trapped nerve', I explained that this terminology is often misleading as the nerves involved are generally not trapped but are irritated and 'sensitised' by inflammatory chemicals released from surrounding tissues or the nerve itself. I also informed him that, unlike his friend, the vast majority of these injuries usually recover with good management and without needing surgery; this was something he was very relieved to hear.

We initially looked at improving his pain management. His GP had prescribed analgesic and anti-inflammatory medication but Sam was not taking these regularly as he believed they were just masking his symptoms. A simple explanation of the action of these drugs and the importance of taking them regularly was enough to change his approach to medication and this resulted in significant reduction of his pain. This provided an ideal opportunity to begin rehabilitating lost function and muscle power at his neck and right upper limb.

Because it is important to progress carefully with 'nerve injuries' (some attempts to abruptly restore restricted spinal movements by forceful manipulation have resulted in catastrophic injuries[7]), I recommended the graded exposure approach. Sam felt happy with my explanation of his problem and was now enthusiastic about exploring movements that could be used to improve his function.

We initially tried some rotational and side-bend movements of his head and neck and established baseline and goal amounts. On returning to clinic he demonstrated significant improvements in these movements. This allowed us to look at gradually strengthening the affected muscles using small mid-range movements in functionally relevant positions, and resistance was introduced using a latex exercise band.

These movements were progressed into the combined patterns of movements needed to carry out his golf swing and once again progressive resistance was added using an exercise band. Sam then progressed onto the practice range with graded golf shot drills right up to his full return to playing golf. We also devised an ongoing exercise programme that he has continued to use to improve his strength and flexibility for golf. He attended his appointments with the neurosurgeon who agreed with Sam that he had progressed well and did not need surgery.

Stephen Robson and Louis Gifford

References

1. *Gifford (2003) In Touch 102:3-15*

2. *Waddell (2003) The Back Pain Revolution, Churchill Livingstone, Edinburgh*

3. *Watson and Kendall (2000) Topical Issues In Pain, 2nd edn, CNS Press Ltd, Falmouth, 111-129*

4. *Hessey S (2005) PPA News 19:33-35*

5. *Frost, Lamb, Doll et al BMJ 2004; 329:708-11*

6. *Gifford, Thacker, Jones 'Physiotherapy & Pain', in McMahon and Koltzenberg (eds) Wall and Melzack's Textbook of Pain, 5th edn, Churchill Livingstone, Edinburgh, 603-617*

7. *Robson (2005) Topical Issues In Pain, 5th edn, CNS Press, Falmouth (in press)*

What all athletes need to know about pain relief medication

Sooner or later the dreaded 'I' word becomes part and parcel of virtually every athlete's vocabulary. If you're exploring your physical limits, or your sport involves the risk of impact, it's only a matter of time before injury strikes, delivering a double whammy. Quite apart from the pain and discomfort of the injury itself, there's the frustration and depression of seeing your hard-earned fitness gains slip away as each inactive day passes. Hardly surprising then that athletes seeking to return to training as soon as possible frequently turn to painkillers, and particularly to anti-inflammatory medication. However, contrary to popular belief, this type of medication can cause potentially serious side effects, and new research indicates that it may even slow down healing and increase susceptibility to injury in the longer term.

If you've ever been injured, you'll be well aware of the associated pain and discomfort that injury brings. But injury also results in inflammation. Sometimes this inflammation is all too apparent (for example a twisted ankle that swells up like a balloon), while at other times it's hidden from view (such as with a shoulder impingement injury, where the inflammation occurs deep in the joint). Inflammation is responsible for much of the pain and discomfort that occurs after injury – but why does it happen?

Inflammation is the body's basic response to injury. When an injury occurs, your body immediately recognises the damaged tissue as 'foreign', and a sequence of complicated and interrelated events are set in motion to defend the body and eradicate the damaged tissue by a process of destruction, followed by renewal.

It's a bit like warfare: if you want your body to be healthy, it must be able to mount an inflammatory response! The general sequence of events following an injury is shown in the box opposite.

The downside of inflammation, however, is that it invariably causes pain and discomfort. Sometimes this can actually be advantageous because the pain forces us to limit the movement in the affected area, and that can help healing; damaged unrepaired tissue is weak tissue and further movement may worsen the injury.

However, there are also times when inflammation can be detrimental, especially when it becomes chronic. For example, joint inflammation due to arthritis may limit motion in a joint, yet maintaining mobility in arthritic joints is crucial for the long-term health of those joints. Although painkillers like codeine and paracetamol can offer pain relief, tackling the inflammation itself is a far more effective strategy, which is where anti-inflammatory medication comes in.

Anti-inflammatory medications are by far the most commonly prescribed medication for pain involving inflammation. They fall into two main categories: steroidal and non-steroidal. Steroidal anti-inflammatories, such as hydrocortisone, are very effective but carry health risks, especially when used for extended periods of time. These risks include skin and blood sugar abnormalities, weakened bones, and even disruption of the body's own steroid production capability, which is why they're only used as a last resort.

By contrast, and as their name suggests, non-steroidal anti-inflammatory drugs (NSAIDs), including aspirin, ibuprofen and diclofenac, among others, don't carry the risks of steroid use and are therefore much preferred by doctors. This also explains why the less potent types of NSAIDs, such as aspirin and ibuprofen, can be freely purchased over the counter. So commonly prescribed and purchased are these drugs that in the UK alone it is estimated that there are between five and eight million regular users!

Inflammation – what happens at tissue level?

1. Damage to tissue *(eg* torn ligament, strain or blow to muscle tissue) allows blood to leak into surrounding tissues. This causes a cascade of biochemical events signalling to the body that injury has occurred, and the acute phase of inflammation begins.

2. One of the first reactions is a widening of the small blood vessels supplying the injured area (vasodilation) resulting in increased blood flow. As well as dilating, these blood vessels also start to become 'leaky' to proteins, allowing proteins in the blood to leak through the vessel wall into the surrounding tissue.

3. The leakage of proteins into surrounding tissue then causes an associated leakage of fluid, which leads to swelling. This swelling often impinges on sensitive nerve endings, causing pain.

4. At this point, neutrophils (a type of white blood cell) exit from the blood vessels into the tissues, followed by monocytes (another type of white blood cell). Their job is to clean out any bacteria and prevent infection at the injury site. Many of the chemicals released during this phase are broken down into hormones, whose role is to tell cells to become active or inactive during this phase of inflammation. Some of these chemicals are called prostaglandins, which can cause pain at the injury site (more about them later).

5. The arrival of the macrophages (yet another type of immune cell) at the injury site signals the beginning of the next phase in the healing process. Macrophages begin to clean up the area through a combination of digesting the broken-down cell parts and secreting enzymes, which break down damaged cells. With all this activity occurring, inflammation (and pain) often peaks at this stage.

6. Once the wound has been successfully cleared of unwanted material it gives way to a process known as granulation, where new tissue is laid down with the help of special cells called fibroblasts and other cells associated with inflammation. Fibroblasts first appear in significant numbers in the wound on the third day post-injury and achieve peak numbers around the seventh day. They are the primary synthetic element in the repair process and are responsible for production of the majority of structural proteins, such as collagen, used during tissue reconstruction. This initial healing phase marks the end of the inflammation phase, although it may take many days or weeks for inflammation to subside completely.

7. The final phase is called 'maturation', whereby the structural proteins in reconstructed tissue are gradually remodelled and strengthened to gain full functionality. This phase can last from a week to a year!

One of the crucial steps in regulating the process of inflammation involves naturally occurring substances called prostaglandins, which are synthesised in our bodies from fatty acids that we consume in our diet. These prostaglandins possess hormone-like properties – *ie* they act as chemical messengers, telling cells what to do, and by so doing play a pivotal role in regulating a number of aspects of our body's chemistry.

There are actually three types, or families, of prostaglandins: series 1 (PG1), series 2 (PG2) and series 3 (PG3 – we don't need to worry about these here). Although PG1 and PG2 prostaglandins are both synthesised from metabolites of linoleic acid (omega-6 – one of the essential fatty acids we eat in our diet), they have very different roles.

- The PG1 family of prostaglandins can be thought of as 'the good guys', helping blood to become less sticky, relaxing blood vessels, improving circulation and lowering blood pressure, enhancing the function of immune T-cells and helping insulin work more effectively in the body. PG1 also helps prevent the release of the fatty acid arachidonic acid (AA) from our cell membranes, where it is normally stored. This is important because AA is the building block from which the PG2 series of prostaglandins are synthesised.
- PG2 prostaglandins are responsible for a number of biochemical 'fight or flight' responses in the body. For example, they increase stickiness of blood (useful for clotting and wound healing), increase blood pressure by stimulating water retention and are responsible for inflammation. But, while they have their role in emergency conditions, under 'normal' conditions many of their effects can be undesirable, which is why they're often referred to as 'the bad guys' of prostaglandins!

NSAIDs work by helping to block the conversion of AA to certain types of PG2s, prostaglandins that orchestrate the process of inflammation, as illustrated graphically in the flow chart, opposite.

How NSAIDs block the inflammation process

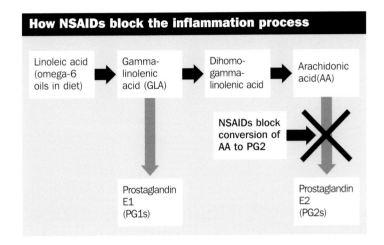

So far, so good, but there's a big problem for sportsmen and women who use NSAIDs, and that is the fact that many of these drugs can play havoc with the delicate lining of the stomach, with the potential to cause such serious gastric problems as ulcers and bleeding.

The risks involved are considerable: in the USA, NSAIDs cause more deaths than bone marrow cancers, asthma, cervical cancer or Hodgkin's disease (cancer of the lymphatic tissues) and about as many as HIV/AIDS[1]. On average, one in every 1,200 patients taking NSAIDs for at least two months will die from gastrointestinal complications – people who would not have died if they had not taken NSAIDs[2]! A large UK study also showed that the risk of NSAID-induced gastric bleeding increases rapidly with age, as does death from complications *(see table, overleaf)*[3].

Of course, no medication is totally without side effects or risks, but the fact is that many people, including sportsmen and women, are completely unaware of the risks relating to NSAIDs.

The reason why many NSAIDs can be so harmful to the stomach lining is to do with the way they block the conversion of AA to PG2s, as illustrated in the diagram.

Before the 1990s, scientists believed that the conversion of AA to PG2s involved a single enzyme called cyclooxygenase.

Table: age-related risk of problems with NSAIDs		
Age range (years)	Chance of GI bleed due to NSAID	Chance of dying from GI bleed due to NSAID
	Risk in any one year is 1 in:	
16-45	2,100	12,353
45-64	646	3,800
65-74	570	3,353
≥ 75	110	647

But then it was discovered that this conversion actually involves two very closely related enzymes – cyclooxygenase 1 and cyclooxygenase 2, or more simply COX-1 and COX-2. However COX-1 and COX-2 have different functions. COX-1 synthesises PG2s that do 'housekeeping' work around a number of organs, such as maintaining the health of the stomach, intestines and kidneys, while COX-2 synthesises the potentially troublesome inflammatory PG2s and oxygen free radicals that enhance inflammation.

The problem with conventional NSAIDs, such as aspirin and ibuprofen, is that they block both enzymes. Yes, they block the production of inflammatory PG2s by COX-2, but the downside is that they exact a heavy price by simultaneously blocking COX-1 and the production of protective PG2s. Some of these protective PG2s are involved in maintaining the integrity of the stomach lining and protecting the stomach wall against the extremely strong acid secreted in the stomach to digest food. Blocking these protective PG2s increases the risk of this acid attacking the stomach wall, leading to such potentially severe gastro-intestinal problems as ulcers and stomach bleeding.

A new generation of NSAIDs

A new generation of NSAIDs, called 'COX-2 inhibitors', has recently appeared on the market. These include such products as rofecoxib, celecoxib and valdecoxib. As the name suggests, these block the COX-2 enzyme, but not the COX-1 enzyme. In other words, they dramatically reduce inflammation without the

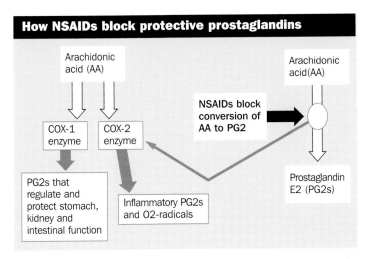

How NSAIDs block protective prostaglandins

harmful gastric effects and risks of conventional NSAIDs. In short, this type of NSAID seems to be the answer to an injured athlete's prayer!

However, some new research on COX-2 inhibitors makes disturbing reading. A group of American scientists examined the effects of COX-2 inhibitors on mice with bone fractures and found that, by comparison with untreated mice, COX-2-treated mice suffered from profoundly compromised bone healing[4]. In particular, the bone nodules that formed (small bony growths that form the first stage of healing) were smaller and did not respond to growth factors that would stimulate bone healing in untreated mice. Moreover, when the COX-2-treated mice were then given a dose of the inflammatory PG2s (which had been blocked by the COX-2 drug), the bone healing process was restored, indicating that these inflammatory PG2s may play an essential role in bone healing.

In addition, several studies have shown that the COX-2 inhibitors celecoxib and rofecoxib either delay or inhibit fracture healing in rats[5,6]; another study found that COX-2 inhibitors decreased the strength of fracture healing at 21 days[7]; and a paper published earlier this year points to evidence that these drugs impair the return of mechanical strength following acute injury to ligaments and tendons as well as bone[8].

Given that it's the blocking of inflammatory PG2 production that seems to be the cause of this delayed healing, eagle-eyed readers out there might be wondering whether traditional NSAIDs (which block both COX-2 and COX-1) also diminish the rate of healing? The answer appears to be 'yes'. A study on rabbits compared the effect of a COX-2 NSAID (celecoxib) with a conventional NSAID (Toradol) on bone healing following a fracture and found no statistical difference[9].

Meanwhile, in a human study, researchers looked at patients who had undergone spinal fusion treatment, where two or more vertebrae are fused together, and discovered that patients who had taken a conventional NSAID (Toradol) were five times less likely to achieve successful union of the vertebrae than those who had taken no NSAID[10].

However, some researchers believe that the extent of healing impairment is far more severe with COX-2 inhibitors. In the COX-2 rat study mentioned above, 253 young rats with broken legs were given either one of two types of COX-2 NSAIDs (Vioxx, Celebrex) or indomethacin, which is a traditional NSAID[5]. The indomethacin-treated rats took a week longer to heal than untreated rats, but the new bone was just as strong. However, rats given Vioxx or Celebrex had not fully healed after two months and the researchers likened the new bone to a 'weakened shell'.

There have been anecdotal reports of impaired bone healing in patients taking traditional NSAIDs for years, but this side effect may have escaped attention because traditional NSAIDs, such as ibuprofen and indomethacin, appear to delay healing instead of blocking it. Interestingly, the report also says aspirin appears to be one of the few NSAIDs that kill pain without this side effect!

Finally, long-term use of some COX-2 NSAIDs may pose other health problems. In 2004, Merck's product Vioxx was withdrawn because of new evidence indicating an increased risk of stroke and heart attack. And just two months ago, Pfizer agreed to suspend sales of another COX-2 drug (Bextra) after US and European regulators said the risk of serious side effects,

Fighting inflammation naturally

After injury, remember the 'RICE' acronym – rest, ice, compression, elevation. Applying ice to the affected area during the early stages of injury is particularly effective at reducing the amount of inflammation and subsequent pain that occurs. A compression bandage around the area can also help.

In chronic injuries, nutritional strategies can also help moderate the degree of inflammation:

- Increasing your intake of omega-3 oils, particularly eicosapentanoeic acid (EPA) found in fish oils (eg salmon, trout, herring, sardines, mackerel, pilchards) helps to block the release of AA from cell membranes and so slows the conversion of AA to inflammatory PG2s. This explains why chronic inflammatory conditions, such as arthritis, are helped by fish oils. Boosting omega-3 oils (found in walnuts, flax and hemp seeds and wheatgerm) will also help because these oils can be transformed into EPA in the body.
- Evening primrose, borage and blackcurrant seed oils contain a rich source of GLA, which can help boost the body's levels of prostaglandin E1, a prostaglandin that suppresses inflammation.
- Antioxidant nutrition is also important, because your body's antioxidant enzymes help to mop up the 'collateral' damage to healthy tissue caused by the release of free radicals in inflammation. Brightly coloured fresh fruits and vegetables are the best source of dietary antioxidants.
- Glucosamine sulphate can be useful for chronically inflamed joints; recent research has indicated that it's at least as effective in reducing pain as ibuprofen!

including a potentially fatal skin allergy, outweighed the benefits. In addition, the US Food and Drug Administration also asked Pfizer to add a 'black box' warning – the strongest possible – to the label of its COX-2 anti-inflammatory painkiller Celebrex.

There is no doubt that NSAIDs can help you return to training and competition more rapidly, and provide effective pain relief in the process. It is also true that the new generation COX-2 inhibiting NSAIDs are much less risky in terms of gastric health. However, every silver lining has a cloud and NSAIDs are no exception! Although more research is needed, there's genuine concern that (aspirin aside) NSAIDs may impair injury healing, especially of bone and ligament. And COX-2 NSAIDs may present more of a problem in this respect than traditional NSAIDs. However, to date there's little evidence about the possible effects of NSAIDs on soft tissue injury healing.

If you're suffering from a soft tissue injury, there's no reason as yet to believe that COX-2 NSAIDs will harm the healing process, and they could be the best option. Injuries involving ligaments or bone are more problematical because some evidence indicates that COX-2 NSAIDs could seriously delay and impair healing, leaving you more vulnerable to re-injury.

On the other hand, if you have a sensitive stomach, a traditional NSAID may cause gastric problems, especially when taken for extended periods of time, and even these NSAIDs appear to delay healing. Ideally you should talk to your GP before rushing into the nearest chemist and buying anti-inflammatories. There are also some very simple guidelines you can use to help reduce inflammation naturally, without resorting to NSAIDs *(see box on page 47)*.

The overall message is that all NSAIDs pose considerable risks and you should use them as a last resort, not a first!

Andrew Hamilton

References

1. *Journal of Rheumatology 1999; 26 Supp 56: 18-24*

2. *Pain 2000; 85: 169-182*

3. *Aliment Pharmacol Ther 1997; 11: 283-91*

4. *Journal of Clinical Investigation 2002; 109(11): 1405-1415*

5. *Journal of Bone and Mineral Research 2002; 17(6): 963-976*

6. *J Bone Joint Surg Am 2004; 86-A(1): 116-23*

7. *Journal of Orthopaedic Research 2003; 21: 670-675*

8. *Sports Med 2005; 35(4): 271-83*

9. *JBJS-Am 2002; 84A(10): 1763-1768*

10. *Spine 1998; 23(7): 834-838*